I0442001

Homegrown Medicinal Herbs

Essential Guide on How to Successfully Grow Medicinal Herbs at Home, Use Natural Remedies & Create DIY Herbal Medicine and Cosmetics

By William Walsworth

1st Edition, March 2016

Table of Contents

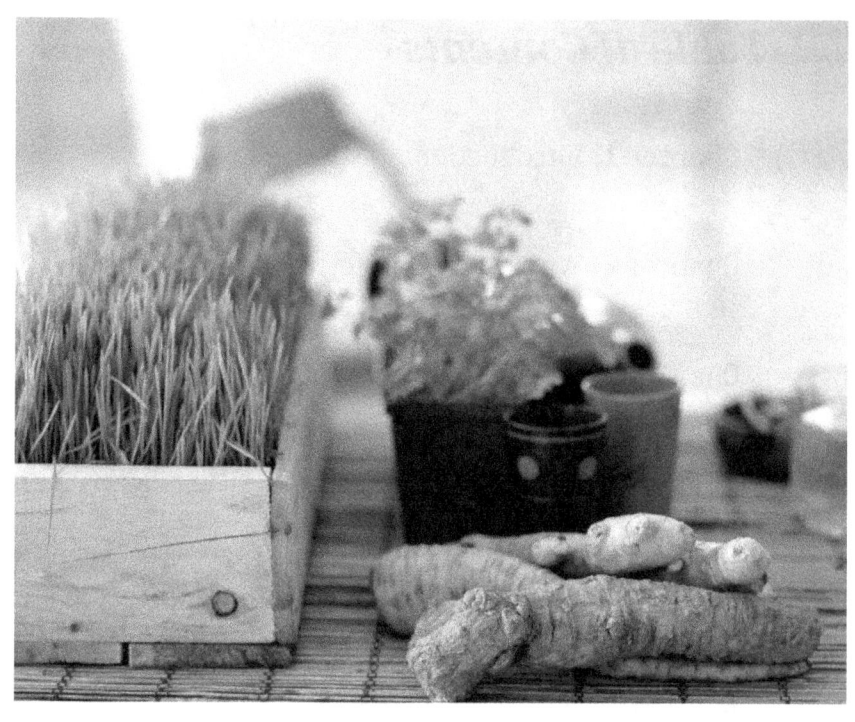

"Plant seeds of happiness, hope, success and love; it will all come back to you in abundance. This is the law of nature."

- Steve Maraboli

Chapter 1: Introduction

Over centuries, the healing power of plants and roots has been acknowledged by many civilizations. The hidden uses of herbs are becoming increasingly popular again, as a natural and healthy counterpart to the traditional word of medicine. More and more people are discovering the healing uses of homegrown natural herbs as an alternative to the corporate industry that is the pharmaceutical world. And by growing these herbs in your own garden, you essentially have your own little natural pharmacy directly in your backyard!

With more and more people choosing technology over spending time in nature, the many stressful situations of the fast-paced life have taken over much of our current modern society. As an opposing force to this modernized stressed life, more people find the appeal and joy in going back to their natural roots. It comes to no surprise that people are choosing to take the slow and sustainable lifestyle over the busy, fast-paced city life. One of the movements that has sprouted from this is the growing group of people seeking to go back to natural remedies and the healing power of natural products: growing their herbs on their own lands, in their own organic and sustainable way. As an essential addition to the 'regular' medicinal world, the healing properties of many natural herbs and plants allow for a cheap and natural alternative. How amazing is it to have your own cabinet of healing plants in your garden that allows you to be completely self-sufficient for solving many common health nuisances?

Getting introduced to herbalism is as much a personal opportunity as it is an opportunity that allows us to become close to our natural roots and knowledge of the land. There are so many species out there that have hidden powers inside them that only few people really have knowledge of and expertise in. This book will allow you to scratch the surface of the many uses of some of the most commonly used herbs in the medicinal and cosmetic world. The knowledge provided in this book will never be a replacement for traditional medicine, but know that they do allow you to become knowledgeable in the healing powers of the herbal world. By learning about herbalism, you are on your way to educating yourself and the people around you about the healing properties of the natural world around you. There is a real chance that some of the plants discussed in this book will already be in your garden or backyard. It are often the most commonly found plants that are overlooked in their multi-purpose abilities. While most people simply use plants for decoration in their garden, some actually have more to them than you would know at first.

With the management of your own small herbal garden, you will be able to provide solutions to your family and community even when you are living self-sufficient and off the grid. Not every person has a pharmacy directly next to their doorstep, and why not use the natural healing powers that are locked inside the plants and herbs we will soon discover? To the common man, the discovery of the herbal world and its many practical applications and uses is often a journey of discovery. When I first uncovered some of the healing powers of herbs, I was probably as blown away by their multipurpose use are you will be after reading this introductory book on herbal healing and cosmetic applications of herbs.

In this book, we'll show you how seven of the most common herbal plants can be used for health and cosmetic purposes. You will be taught the basics about the plants themselves, as well as how to be able to grow them easily in your own backyard or other garden area. After uncovering some of the most essential healing purposes, we will consider whether the plant has some possible cosmetic uses as well. You could think about using the plant as a resource for making soap, shampoo or other bathroom products. These products can be used by yourself, or could even be sold at a reasonable price to others if you are willing to take that route.

However, it is also essential to pinpoint the possible dangers and caveats of the many uses the herbs will have. Not every herbal solution is completely without danger, just like the medication is in your local pharmacy. It is therefore very important to consider some potential dangers of using the herbal products. However, do not let this discourage you as a beginner to get into herbalism. With normal use of the plants under review in this book, there is little that could really be considered 'dangerous'. However, I like to take the risks into consideration as well, thus making it essential to also include potential dangers of the uses these herbs have.

Get ready for the first major investment in your future herbal garden: learning about all of the essentials of herbalism and its many practical uses. In this introductory book we'll talk exclusively about seven commonly used herbs. This allows you to become familiarized with the word of herbalism as a natural alternative to the traditional medicinal world. The herbs discussed in this book have been chosen carefully and most of them have also personally helped me to live a healthier lifestyle.

Having a biology background, the world of herbs and plants has always intrigued me and I am more than excited to uncover some of the knowledge I have built up over the years. I am sure many of you will be able to resonate with the natural healing powers of some common herbs that will be discussed. From lavender to thyme, and lemon balm to basil: the herbal word is filled with opportunities and a sea of in-depth practical knowledge. Please follow me on the journey to learning about the seven most commonly used herbs and their natural applications in health and cosmetics.

Chapter 2: Why Medicinal Herbs?

There are many valid reasons why people would consider growing medicinal herbs themselves. Whether you live in in the suburbs of a large city, or perhaps somewhere in the middle of the countryside, in America or Asia, Europe or Australia: the benefits of herbal remedies are always the same. Depending on the herbs you are interested in growing, you will be able to solve a whole range of small medical nuisances, as well as being able to produce your own healing cosmetic products. By growing your own herbs, you will be able to achieve self-sufficiency and become less dependent on expensive pharmacy drugs, you will come closer to nature by using only homegrown natural products, you will learn invaluable lessons about the uses of common plants and herbs, and you will ultimately become healthier and happier from using the end products you will produce, mainly because of the many types of healing powers many of the herbs naturally have.

We must see natural remedies such as the medicinal herbs covered in this book as a supplement to traditional pharmaceuticals, not just as a full replacement. It is very important to always consult a doctor when you are experiencing a serious medical condition or a long-term medical problem. However, for simple health solutions, including common problems like headaches, muscle pain or a simple flu, it might be very helpful to try out some naturally produced herbal remedies. If these common household health problems do not go away after applying both traditional and natural remedies, consult your local health center for a checkup. I cannot stress enough the importance of the need for professional healthcare if you are sick. Medicinal herbs can help you get rid of simple health problems and nuisances only.

Another reason for growing herbs lie in some of their other common uses. Herbal plants are also a great basic source of homemade cosmetic products. You can think of shampoos, soaps, perfumes, deodorants, and many more related bathroom products. As a natural alternative to the chemical junk that is processed in traditional cosmetics, herbal plants offer an amazing healthy natural alternative to the products you will find in your local supermarket that are often full of ingredients we cannot even pronounce the names of. Cosmetics in particular have large companies behind them dominating the market. Small-scale natural produce is very rarely found if they are offered at all. Organically and locally produced items are however on the rise, and joining the green homegrown movement is a great opportunity. All you need is your own backyard, the right type of plants, and a simple ingredients list to get you on track for making these products in your kitchen.

Most common medicinal herbs, at least those covered in this book, are easy to grow and do not require much effort to produce at all. With the basic step-by-step system outlined for you, everyone practically applying the growth methods in this book is able to produce a nice harvest of herbs in their own backyard. You don't need a hundred acres or even a dozen acres to be a successful herbalist. The whole idea of homemade medicinal herbs revolves around the concept of using a relatively small piece of land to efficiently produce hand-made and locally grown herbal products.

For some people, gardening and growing their own herbs is merely a passion and a way to spend free time. However, most aspiring herbalists are seeking a long-term natural alternative to sometimes expensive medicinal products. Why buy painkillers, anti-inflammatory pills or even soaps and shampoo's when you can take pride and joy in producing your own natural alternatives right where you live? With the aid of the extensive step-by-step processes and explanations in this book you will be able to understand the uses and caretaking processes for useful types of herbal plants a little better. The natural world has blessed us with the unique opportunity to use the healing powers of these herbs to improve our lives. Our co-existence with the living things around us has allowed these species to flourish and adapt: our increased cultivation efforts have strengthened the healing powers and uses of most herbs over thousands of years. Therefore, to seek the true reasons why we must learn about medicinal herbs we must take a brief look into the history of their applications. It is true that we have lost some, if not most of our knowledge on these natural remedies because of the introduction of medicine in pill-form. Health solutions came from nature by default.

Chapter 3: A Brief History of Medicinal Herbs

Looking back in time, we see a natural co-evolution between humans and the plants that are useful to them. Wherever societies blossom, there are certain herbal species that blossom together with them. Knowledge of uses of certain plants are passed down generations, and only in recent times a significant shift has happened. We have become somewhat disconnected from our natural roots and have generally resorted to synthetic pharmaceutical solutions as opposed to using the natural medicinal powers of herbal plants. With the rise of modern-day medical facilities, our collective knowledge of herbalism is on the decline. Only very recently a movement sprouted that is seeking to take the more sustainable path and resort back to traditional herbal methods.

Our Medicinal Roots...

When we look at the timeline of human existence, there really has not been a moment we did not apply some type of natural solution to our health problems.

Ever since we humans were hunter-gatherers, we have sought natural products, especially herbal plants, and used them to treat many types of health problems. Over time, the knowledge of the most useful and common herbs became institutionalized into our culture, and generation upon generation the knowledge has been passed on. The earliest evidence of medicinal plant usage dates back to the Paleolithic era, which was roughly 60,000 years ago. This long history clearly shows our deeply rooted connection with the healing powers of herbs. The first written evidence is Mesopotamian and dates back over 5,000 years. The fact that over 100 herbs are mentioned in the Bible shows how important they must have been to the medicinal cultures several millennia ago. It was only until the Middle Ages that more books and texts on the topic became common, and this was also the period that the first extreme detailed descriptions (including biologically accurate drawings) showed up. Most of the knowledge was kept in monasteries, again showing a clear historical connection between religion and herbalism knowledge. The religious beliefs often where a great method to keep the knowledge from fading and embedding herbalism into religion allowed for consistent passing on of most of the knowledge for most of the historical time.

The Beginning of a Decline

The first real turnaround in popularity of herbal medicinal solutions came during the period where the black plague started to take a significant death toll within medieval societies. It soon became apparent to the medieval people that some of the healing properties in the plants were not going to stop them from getting this horrible disease, and the overall trust in herbs as a healing method slowly eroded, taken over by solutions that were a lot more painful to the patients.

At times where bloodletting and other obscure medical practices where the norm, colonization of the America's did allow for a small revival of the Western knowledge with regards to plant uses. The Native Americans brought some of the century-old knowledge of indigenous plant species over to the colonists and the newly acquired knowledge was (often informally) spread across most of Europe. Nevertheless, the coming of modern medical solutions was near and herbalism was pushed to a background position and more commonly referred to as an alternative to most of the modern recommended pharmaceuticals.

Herbalism During Modern Times

As said, the modern-day pharmaceutical industry has more than taken over herbalism as a common solution to health problems. During the Great Depression, a time in the 1930's where economic decline and poverty where common issues, the American government even began to put nation-wide bans on the practice of herbalism. Although herbalism has always been one of the foundations upon which the human race has thrived, the concept of homegrown medicinal herbs is a fairly new concept in our modernized societies. The rise of the sustainable and green movements, as well as the increased call for providing medicinal solutions when regular pharmaceuticals no longer offer a satisfactory solution, has allowed some window of opportunity to open again for herbal medicine. With more people seeking alternatives to the big corporations and more people wanting to go back to organic, green natural produce, herbalists have slowly regained their importance among a growing core group of people within the Western society.

However, the importance of herbal medicine is more than clearly visible on a global scale. It is estimated by the World Health Organization that well over 80 percent of the global population is using some form of herbal medicine in their daily lives. Plant-based medicines, both with and without prescriptions, are very common and treatments with these type of herbal products are on the rise. These herbal products are often praised as a viable alternative due to their low possibility for negative side-effects and their low production costs. As we will see in the upcoming chapters, the possibilities of herbal medicine, but also their other uses, are virtually limitless.

Chapter 4: Lavender

In this section, we'll cover all the ins and outs of one of the most common herbs used for many medicinal purposes. The lavender plant, also known as lavandula, is a plant that can be found all across the world. The most widely found species is the *Lavandula angusttifolia*, which is the Latin name for this plant that belongs to the mint family called *Lamiaceae*. Lavender plants are commonly used as culinary herbs, while the extraction of their essential oils is generally used for medicinal purposes, basically serving as a natural remedy alternative to some of the more common health-related problems.

Introduction to Lavender

Lavender is easily recognized by its bright purple flower and long, thin green stem. The nectar from the flower is loved by nectar-loving creatures (such as bees) and these are almost always found in their direct surroundings. Lavender does not only have a wide range of practical purposes, it is also a great addition to any type of garden because of its bright colors and pivotal role in the natural biological cycle.

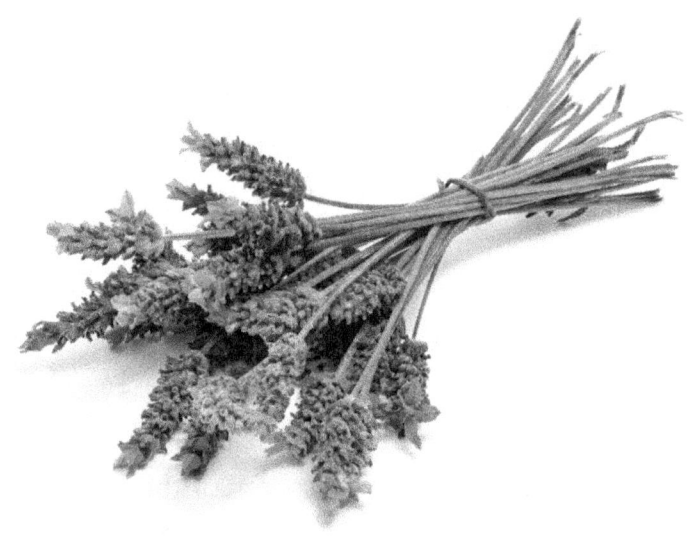

There are many types of different subspecies to be found in the *Lamiaceae* family, and their most common differences include the shape of their leaves, of which the hairs include most of the essential oils. The most cultivated species have these hairs, but there are also subspecies who do not. The color as well as the overall shape of the flower might differentiate slightly. You can find blue, yellow, blackish purple, as well as violet variations, each with their own slight differences in flower shape. English lavender (*L. angusttifolia*), as shown in the image above, is the most commonly applied and cultivated variation. Other common species variations (*L. stoechas, L. lanata & L. dendata*) are generally referred to as Spanish or French lavender.

How to Grow

Growing lavender is actually not that complicated. These plants, at least the cultivated version, are widely available in your local garden shop, whether they are sold in the form of seeds or (semi-)full grown plants. Lavender is a plant with only little requirements, so growing your plant will be possible for beginners without any serious issue. The following easy 5-step process is the recommended procedure. An explanation will be provided for each step below.

1. Soil preparation
2. Nursery pot preparation
3. Planting your herb
4. Herb maintenance
5. Harvesting

Step 1: Soil preparation

First of all, you want to find the perfect location for your lavender plants. Find a well-lit location in your garden to place your plants. If you prefer to grow them in a pot or other container-type location, always ensure that the soil has adequate drainage possibilities. The main idea is that lavender roots should not get overhydrated as they are highly sensitive to excess water in their system. Next, we want to check the correct pH-level of your soil. This should be close to neutral (pH-level of 7, preferably within the range of 6.7-7.3) and can be easily checked with pH-strips you can get at your local garden facility. If you find that the levels of your soil are good, dig a small hole in the ground that is just big enough for the roots of the plant to fit into.

Prepare your soil with a pre-made mixture of two handfuls of round stone and half a cup of a mixture of lime and manure (or similar fertilizer). The small round stone is there to aid with water drainage. The mixture of lime and manure (fertilizer) makes sure that the initial plant growth is supported and that the soil is alkalized correctly. Apply both pre-made mixtures to the bottom of the small hole you made for the lavender. Cover the applied mixture up with a thin layer of regular soil (we do not want the roots of the plant to come into contact with the mixtures).

Step 2: Nursery pot preparation

The lavender plant you bought should be in a nursery pot, and it is recommended to water the plant in the nursery pot before doing anything else with it. When it is adequately watered, the plant is ready to be pruned. Carefully and lightly prune your lavender along the sides. This stimulates the internal air circulation and is an important growth stimulant as well. It will also help with a common problem during the lavender's growth, which is the prevention of wooding within the center of the stem. Lavender has the tendency to wooden up at the base of the stem and pruning helps in avoiding this problem.

If you are satisfied with your pruning activities (don't remove too much, or the pant might die), it is time to take it out of the nursery pot. Prepare the lavender's roots. Remove the plant from the pot and continue to remove all soil from the roots. The introduction of a new soil environment helps with the plant's growth and adaptation process. Therefore this step is crucial in long-term growth success.

Step 3: Planting your herb

Place the roots into the prepared hole in the soil, above the stone/lime/fertilized mixed soil you put in before. Roots should not come into contact with the mixture. Fill up the empty extra space with normal soil, patting it lightly into place above the stem of the lavender.

Make sure that you leave around 35 inches (90cm) of space in between individual lavender plants for optimal growth and air circulation possibilities. Planting should be done with care and with the least amount of potential damage to the plant as possible. Always make sure to not water your plant too much after you placed it in another location.

Step 4: Herb maintenance

Fertilize the soil with earlier explained mixture once a year. The fertilization process ideally is done in early springtime. An optional extra summer fertilization in the summertime is possible. Do this by preparing a fish or seaweed-extract mixture onto the soil of the plant (maximum two times).

Lavender is generally a low-maintenance plant and therefore requires little help in terms of its growth after you have planted it in your garden. Most importantly, there should be very limited watering of the plant – too much dampness near the roots will kill the plant quicker than periods of drought of freezing. The most common cause of death for the lavender plant is the fact that people are too enthusiastic with watering them. Especially lavender is very sensitive to excess hydration. To avoid problems with overwatering, make sure that the soil is completely dry between watering sessions. If you grow your lavender in a pot or container, the best option is to apply a drainage option to prevent that too much water will start to accumulate at the bottom of your pot or container, consequently overhydrating your plants.

Another issue is the prevention of weeds. An easy method to prevent unwanted weeds to grow near your plant is to apply a thin layer of mulch near the stem's base. Examples of good mulch include gravel, shells, or sand. An additional benefit of applying this layer is prevention of any frost issues during the wintertime. Don't make the layer too thick to ensure that the plant is still able to hydrate.

Prune your lavender once a year in the spring. Don't be shy when pruning your plant: about 1/3 of the entire plant should be removed. This encourages new growth and prevents any type of unwanted sprawling of the lavender. However, don't go overboard with pruning either as this might possibly kill the plant. Use common pruning shears or perhaps a hedge trimmer for the pruning process.

Step 5: Harvesting

The optimal harvest time for your lavender is when you notice the bottom flowers of the plant are beginning to open themselves. This ensures that the plant is fresh and the essential oils inside the plant have accumulated most of the beneficial properties.

Cutting the flowers should be done near the stem's base, as close as possible to the foliage. Make a straight and clean cut to ensure your final product will not be damaged in any way.

You could opt to dry the plant in large bundles, ideally around one hundred individual plants with a tight rubber band holding them together. Keep the dried plants indoors in a warm and dark part of the house. Suspend your lavender upside down for about two weeks. Use a nail to keep them hanging steadily in one place.

The essential oils can be extracted through a process of steam distillation. You could either set up a semi-professional distillation system, or simply extract the oils using a pan and some heat and water. However, a distillation setup is the preferred option because of the purity of the distilled flower extracts, although it will have some upfront investment costs. There are plenty of guides on the internet to help you with this process. I recommend following several video tutorials available on YouTube or other video websites to get a basic idea of the steam distillation process.

We will not go into the details of the distillation process in this book, but there are plenty of free resources out there that can aid you in this process. If you have a hard time understanding the requirements and processes, ask your local chemistry teacher or advisor (someone with laboratory experience) to help you out with the setup. A semi-professional distillation setup like this will cost you about $500, and can be used with most of the herbal products you are going to produce. Any type of essential oil will be produced with the process of distillation, so consider it as a worthwhile investment if you want to get serious within the homemade herbal products world.

Generally, you will need the following basic distillation items for your needs:

- One two-neck round bottom distillation flask (1 liter)

- One 300-mm condenser (Allihn or Liebig)

- Oil can be collected in a Clevenger trap

- A heating mantle

- A variable voltage transformer

- A ring stand and three clams for support

- Two 5-foot lengths of 3/8-inch plastic tubing (for circulation of the water through the condenser)

- An adapter to connect the tubing to your home water supply

- One large rubber or glass stopper for the large flask

Health Applications

Lavender oil has a wide range of beneficial applications. There are over a dozen known health applications, most of which are related to applying lavender oil to the skin. Below you can find a brief discussion of the most common medicinal applications of lavender oil.

Aches and pain: If your muscles are worn out after a long day of hard work, a soothing bath with some lavender oil will help you reduce the feeling of muscle or tissue pressure and instantly relieve them.

Fever reduction: For kids suffering from a severe fever, putting a few lavender oil drops in water at body temperature provides the ideal bath to aid with the effects of fever. Additionally, it is very helpful for allowing them to sleep better that night as well. So it is preferred if you prepare a tepid lavender bath for your child before bedtime.

Acne and eczema treatment: Lavender oil is strongly antibacterial and applying it to the skin reduces harmful bacteria and moisturizes it. Applying the oil to the skin helps prevent secretion of certain body fluids (such as sebum) that are food for bacterial growth and a breeding ground for infections in the upper skin. Especially children suffering from eczema are benefited by the regular use of lavender oils on the areas of the skin that itch and have become dry.

Earache soothing: For any type of infected or irritated ear, lavender has always proven the most ideal solution to relieving ear pain. Take a droplet pipet and slowly massage a few drops of lavender oil onto the skin around the ears. This also works with applying to the throat area: the sensations of pain throughout the face will reduce and the healing process is consequently speeded up.

Burn effect reduction: The soothing effect of the oil on the skin helps the treatment of minor burns and instantly relieves any type of pain caused by the burn itself. Furthermore, it helps to heal the affected skin area over time. Just a few drops of lavender oil are enough.

Reduces stress in muscle and mind: Lavender oil also as an avid stress-reducer. Whilst generally used in hot or tepid water baths, the application of a few drops of oil onto the forehead, temples and neck reduce headache effects and induce calmness of the mind and head muscles. It is recommended to also use a piece of cloth or a towel, sprinkled with lavender oil, to apply to the facial area in case of a headache or moment of severe stress.

Fighting motion sickness: When travelling, apply a mixture of lavender oil, sage and rosemary to your pulse points to help you reduce nausea. Pulse points are specific areas of the body where the heart beating can easily be detected. See if you can detect some veins or beating of your heart in your own body: these generally fall under the 'pulse point' category. Easy pulse point herbal oil application can be done on the wrist or neck.

Heals cuts and bruises: Applying the oil to a paper cut or a painful blue bruised area helps to remove the burning sensation. Additionally, the strong anti-bacterial properties in the oil reduces the chance of infections to develop near the affected areas.

Sleep inducement: When applying only a few droplets of oil on your pillow before sleep, you will experience a calm and well-rested sleep. Deep rest can be very important for people who have sleeping problems, kids, or both. Speaking from experience, it can also be helpful to bathe children who are hyperactive in a lavender oil bath. The calmness-inducing properties of the herb really are helpful.

Menstrual cramp reduction: For the females out there that know what it is like to have severe monthly cramps, applying some lavender oil near the cramped areas can really help with some pain relief. Alternatively, use a hot compress that is induced with oil on the surface.

Fights off insects (including scabies): As it turns out, the insects that are after your body for blood and other stinging or buzzing-related activities, also really dislike the smell and taste of lavender oil. Get some water and induce it with oil, and apply it to the neck, feet and arms. These the areas most prone to attract unwanted insects. Keep a soaked cotton cloth with you to make sure your entire evening will become insect-free. This also works great with scabies, tiny mites that like to borrow themselves into the skin. If left untreated these creates could even be life-threatening, so a pinch of lavender oil is very welcome.

Fights Shingles: Also referred to as Herpes Zoster, these tiny painful infected skin areas are the cause of an annoying virus. Whilst generally these rashes are not dangerous, they can be very annoying and painful. The healing properties of lavender can help reduce pain and speed up the healing process.

Treats Sinusitis: When inhaling the vapor of lavender oil, chronic Sinusitis can be treated effectively. The infection will quickly be gone when you make some steaming lavender water for yourself. Also, the pain along the healing process will be reduced significantly.

Cosmetic Applications

As we uncovered already, the anti-bacterial properties as well as the skin treatment properties, allow for the use of lavender oil in a variety of different cosmetic products. There is a wide range of products using lavender essence and you can surely think of some uses already yourself. One scientific study by Michalun spoke of lavender as a product that is *"anti-allergenic, anti-inflammatory, antiseptic, antibacterial, antispasmodic, balancing energizing, soothing, healing, toning and stimulating"*. Treating minor wounds, skin problems and sunburns are just some of the uses of lavender oil.

Lavender is an avid candidate for one of the best products to treat minor health issues, anything from hay fever to beestings can be treated. Remove lip balm, ointments, painkillers, soaps, shampoos and much more products from your drawers and replace it with a minor amount of lavender oil applied to the area of your choice. The cosmetic world has found lavender to be in up to 20 different product groups, all the way from bath gels to lotions.

For the people that enjoy tea, extracts of the flower can also be transformed in a delicious lavender tea product. An area that is especially recommendable is the treatment of muscle pain and sub-surface skin care. The use of only few drops of oil can help speed up the haling process quickly. Just consider some of the healing properties described earlier and you can surely think of some products to replace in your bathroom drawer. Get rid of those industrial things, use natural solutions and be just as happy and healthy.

Potential Dangers

As with many things in life, the use of herbal plants is not completely without risk or potential dangers. Let us discuss some of the things you must consider when using products originating from the lavender plant. First of all, it is very important to NEVER directly ingest lavender oil. It is a product that can only be applied on inhaled via aromatherapy (or similar therapies). When ingested directly, serious health problems might occur. Symptoms include blurry vision or burning of the eyes, breathing problems, vomiting and diarrhea.

It is not recommended to use lavender while pregnant or breastfeeding. While there is no direct scientific evidence of negative effect for these risk groups, the lack of knowledge in this field requires the governmental agencies (at least those in America) to advice the prevention of use for these risk groups specifically. Furthermore, young boys should avoid the long-term use of lavender due to possibly harmful hormonal side-effects. Studies found that use in this target group could cause pre-puberty skin problems. Skin problems can also be found with people having a hyper sensitive skin. This group can have possible allergic reactions to the lavender oil.

For people that are about to get surgery, it is recommended to stop using lavender products at least two weeks prior to the anesthesia procedure. This procedure, together with the medication used during and after surgery, can have effects on the central nervous system when lavender products are involved.

Chapter 5: Thyme

Another herbal plant with a variety of different practical uses is the Thyme plant. This herb can be used in two different forms, either by their essential oils or their leaves. While the oil is mostly used for medicinal purposes, the leaves are applied as an edible taste-maker for culinary purposes. Lastly, thyme is rather popular as an ornamental plant as well.

Introduction to Thyme

Thyme, their most commonly used species being the *Thymus vulgaris* (no really, it's not vulgar at all), is part of the mint family *Lamiaceae*. Thyme is a close relative to oregano, another herb that is known for its culinary use. The uses of thyme go way back to the ancient civilizations. Ancient Egyptians used the herb in their embalming process, whilst the ancient Greeks used them in bathhouses. However, the Romans popularized the herb by using it as a tastemaker in cheeses and alcoholic beverages.

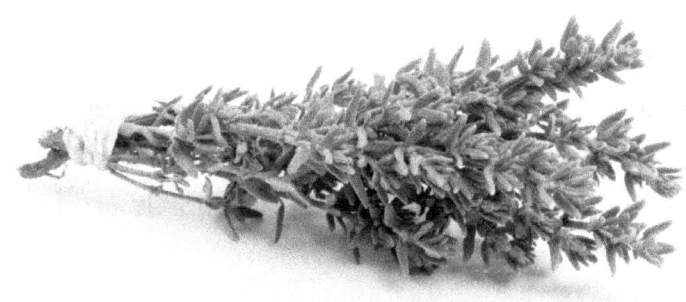

The working ingredient that is sought after by medicinal herbalists is the substance called *thymol*, which composites about 20 to 50% of the essential oil. If you ever took Listerine mouthwashes, chances are you washed your mouth with some thyme, since the herb is strongly antiseptic in nature. This antibacterial property makes it an ideal candidate for many medicinal purposes.

How to Grow

Thyme thrives in hot, sunny places with a soil that is well-drained. The nice thing about thyme is that it is really sturdy and can grow pretty much anywhere the sun shines. It really is the anchor of the herbal garden due to the fact that it remains green throughout the seasons. Just like lavender, the best moment to plant thyme is in the springtime. However, the planting process is a little different. Thyme does not necessarily need a lot of watering, but it is recommended to water them enough during the planting process. When you first place your thyme plants in your garden, make sure the soil is well-drained. It is possible to use a similar soil fertilizer mixture as with lavender.

Generally, the only difference from the lavender growth process is the fact that thyme can be grown close together and thrives in the full sun. The herb needs little extra care, apart from a slight pruning process once a year in the springtime (as much as one third of the total plant can be pruned). Always prune the plant at the points where you can see new growth starting, after all the entire idea of pruning is to stimulate this new growth process within the plant. If you want to ensure the thyme stays bushy and flourishing, you can clip the tips off regularly until the first frost period comes. Thyme thrives in drier soil, no need for constant watering. It will easily survive on rainwater alone.

In cold climate weather, it is important to keep the thyme from freezing. You can do this by applying a thin layer of sand or gravel onto the soil. Additionally, extra protection in the form of pine boughs to cover the thyme with can help with keeping the plant safe from any frost issues in heavy winter.

One problem during the maintenance process is the danger of spider mites. Especially during dry weather, these mites can be a nuisance. An easy and organic method to get rid of these critters is to spray them with a strong stream of water, or alternatively wipe all the leaves of the plants off with a wet sponge. Remove any type of leaves or plants that are too heavily infested. Next, get a sprayer with some rosemary oil (or a pesticide based on this herbal oil) and spray the plants lightly. Alternatively, use a soap solution. Spiders love these mites as well, so a garden that favors spiders can help reduce the probability of getting spider mites in the first place.

For harvesting time, the process is extremely simple. Just take what you need from the plant when you need it. In practice, it is very difficult to overharvest considering the amount that is required for most essential oil extraction processes or food recipes. This can even be done in wintertime, the weather conditions are not relevant for the harvesting period. After cutting what you need, separate the leaves from the stem and discard the stem itself or put it on your compost heap. The leaves are what we are after for the essential oils, or we can simply use them as is for their culinary and aromatic purposes.

Consider preserving thyme in a variety of ways. You could dry them in bundles (see image at the start of this chapter), refrigerate or freeze them, or alternatively preserve them in oil or vinegar. The essential oils are extracted by (steam) distillation. Expose the plant to concentrated steam to evaporate the oils. Just like any distillation process back in chemistry-class, water and oil will not mix, so any vapor that is caught can be easily separated. There are plenty of instructional videos and guides that go into the details of distillation of essential oils. This book will not go over these processes in detail, but the basic idea is to invest in a simple distillation set-up. Please refer back to the lavender distillation process for the needed items and basic directions where to find information on the topic.

Health Applications

Whilst thyme is generally a loved culinary product and tastemaker in many recipes, it also has a range of health benefits. These benefits are generally attained in the form of essential thyme oil. Let us take a look at some of the core benefits of the herb for your health.

Lowers blood pressure: The working components in thyme aid in the process of reducing the heart rate when having high blood pressure. Studies have also found that the herb might be responsible for lowering cholesterol in the blood. A great way to make sure your cardiovascular system is benefited by thyme is to use it as a replacement of salt in your food. High-salt intake is a serious problem that is caused by many of today's food products that are either containing excess amounts of salt or sugar. These additives can harm the body when used in large amounts. Thyme as a tastemaker really helps to reduce the amount of overall salt intake when using it as a replacement product.

Stops coughing or throat irritations: The prime use of the essential oil from the thyme's leaves is used as cough medicine. The essential oils in thyme help to loosen up the lung tissue. They are thus also very helpful for other-lung related problems. In combination with something like an ivy leave, thyme oil can also help fight symptoms of bronchitis.

Immunity booster: Thyme is a great source of vitamins as well, thus it can be of great help as a replacement for vitamin supplements. The leaves of the thyme plant are jam-packed with vitamin C, which is an essential component in your everyday diet. Also, it provides a good chunk of your daily vitamin A intake, which is great for your body and overall health. You think that is all? Nope. Thyme is a source of manganese, iron, copper and fibers. Thyme can also be great as a remedy when you feel an upcoming flu or nasal problem (such as a common cold). Overall, a perfect immunity boost for your body.

Anti-bacterial and antiviral properties: The strong disinfecting properties of thyme allow it to be a helpful herb for improving your indoor air quality and thereby your overall respiratory health. If there is any type of mold rowing indoors, a little bit of thyme oil can easily get rid of it. One of the working components of thyme oil, *thymol*, holds strung anti-fungal properties that allow you to get rid of mold once and for all. The same properties let thyme oil also be a good natural pesticide and insecticide in your garden. It gets rid of many bacteria, viruses, mosquitos, flies, but also larger critters like mice and larger rodents.

Enhances the mood and overall well-being: Another active substance in thyme called *carvacrol* is a therapeutic substance that can actively alter the neurons in your brain. Studies found that this substance has the capacity to alter the mood when used as an aromatic substance in thyme oil within the home. When using thyme oil regularly indoors, the studies suggest that it is possible that your overall mood and feelings get a little positive boost as well. Thyme really can literally make you a happier person!

Disinfects and provides aroma: A last property of thyme oil is the disinfectant abilities of the product. There is a reason that a wide variety of cosmetic products uses thyme oil as an ingredient. The strong smell, as well as the anti-bacterial properties, allow it to be used in a range of different cosmetics. The next section will go into a little more detail about this. Furthermore, thyme leaves are a commonly used ingredient in many mean and fish dishes. The herb is edible and the strong odor and taste really spices up many dishes. Culinary use of thyme is great with pasta, rice or pesto-related dishes. Also, improve your diet with thyme in seafood, which is good for the cardiovascular system and thus healthy for the heart.

Cosmetic Applications

There are many products in the world of cosmetics that find thyme oil to be a useful ingredient. Mainly due to its strong aromatic and anti-bacterial and anti-fungal properties, dentists love the product in mouthwash and thyme oil is one of the most commonly used ingredients in it. Create your own mouth wash easily with this natural disinfectant. A quick homemade recipe for mouthwash:

Ingredients:

- Baking soda (2 teaspoons)
- Warm water (0.5 cup)
- Peppermint essential oil (2 drops)
- Tea tree oil (1-2 drops)
- Thyme essential oil (2 drops)
- Neem oil (1 teaspoon)
- Honey (1 teaspoon)

Mix the warm water with baking soda, peppermint and tea tree oil and stir them slowly but thoroughly. Add neem oil, honey and thyme oil while you are doing the mixing. It's as simple as that. When mixed thoroughly enough, your mouthwash will be ready instantly.

There is also a big market for thyme oil in skin-care products (especially the organic versions of them). Thyme is simply added by large retailers in these skin products to enhance the smell and to improve the disinfecting properties of the mixture. Furthermore, natural deodorants commonly add thyme oil for its aromatic purposes. Their smell combined with their anti-bacterial properties make it an ideal natural additive in deodorants.

Potential Dangers

It is advised that thyme oil should not be directly applied to the skin itself, since it may cause sensitization. First, dilute the concentrated thyme oil with another type of natural oil, otherwise it will be too strong. As you could see from the ingredient list for homemade mouthwash, only a few droplets of concentrated thyme oil are plenty. This means that the oil is very strong and potent, and therefore can be dangerous in large amounts. Also, you have to make sure that you do not have any thyme oil allergies, so first use a small amount to test if this is the case.

It is advised to never take in the oil internally, as it may cause a range of dangerous health issues. Always dilute the product before use. Risks of direct internal use include nausea and dizziness, vomiting, diarrhea and muscle issues. Long-term intake of pure essential oil may damage the heart, lungs and overall balance of the body temperature, as well as stimulate the thyroid gland. This is also one of the main reasons that people suffering from hyperthyroidism should not use any type of thyme oil-related products at all.

Furthermore, risk groups that should avoid thyme oil are people who have high blood pressure, pregnant females, infants and young children. The reason behind this is that thyme oil affects the blood circulation process, which may cause health issues within these risk groups.

Chapter 6: Marigold

In this section, we'll cover one of the prettiest flowers I have growing in my own garden, the shiny orange and round-shaped Marigold flower. Especially during the summertime, these flowers are a real gem in any garden and certainly will impress your visitors if you maintain them correctly. They are easy to grow and offer a wide range of health benefits.

Introduction to Marigold

Marigold, or as biologists like to refer to it '*Calendula officinalis*', is a plant that is commonly found in gardens in Europe (especially England), but also thrives well in the moderate or warm climates of America. While their origin is found in southern Europe, the cultivation process has led this flower mainly to be grown as a common garden herb.

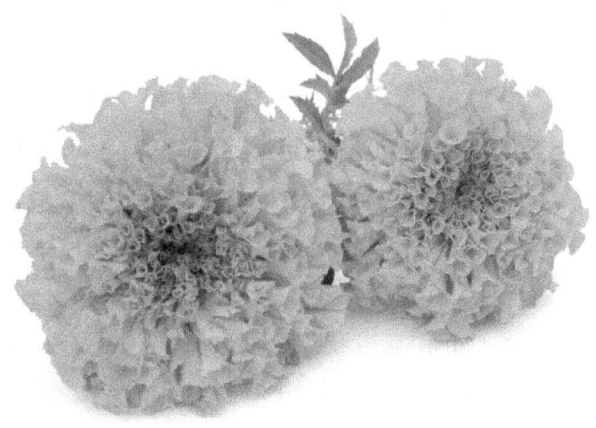

The plant is strongly aromatic and can grow up to 31 inches (80cm) in height during summertime. They have leaves that can grow up to 7 inches (17cm) long, but are mostly grown for their beautiful flowers. While thriving in most gardens, the marigold flower is short-lived and treated as an annual product. Especially in the cold winters, the plant tends to die during the wintertime, which is why most people using them as herbs prefer to harvest them before the first frost kicks in.

How to Grow

The growth process of the marigold flower is slightly different from the other herbs expanded upon in this book, mainly due to the fact that the flower will generally not survive the wintertime. The annual nature of this plant and the strong sensitivity of the marigold flower to cold temperatures, means there should be several considerations for the growing process.

The first step, and this is especially important for people living in colder regions of the planet, is to determine which growth zone you live in. For people in the United States, this growth zone as been determined based on which state you live in. The zones range from the extremely hostile and cold 'Zone 1' (Alaska) to the hot and humid 'Zone 13' (Puerto Rico, Hawaii). Anything in between is determined by the 1 to 13 zoning scale, most of the states falling under Zone 3 up until Zone 10. Consult the United States Department of Agriculture (USDA) website to determine which zone you live in.

Overall, marigold is a hardy and sturdy plant (apart from the issues with frost). It is best to plant them right after the last frosty day. Preferably, do this on a cloudy day or during the early morning, as the soil transplant for marigold can cause a heat shock. Whereas thyme thrives in scorching hot summer days, marigold doesn't mind a little shade every once in a while. They are sun worshippers generally, but thrive in places with up to 20% shade as well. You must make sure that sunlight can be obtained by the flowers, because in fully shaded areas they will die.

Marigold can be both located in flowerbeds and in your herbal section of your garden. Regardless of the container, pot, flowerbed (or soil) they are grown in, place the plants at least 2 to 3 feet apart to ensure airflow and soil nutrient uptake. Also, this ensures that each individual flower will have plenty of sunlight for themselves. When planting the flower, loosen the soil and dig to about 6 inches (15cm). It is recommended to use a hand aerating tool or a hoe to break up the soil and ensure that oxygen is taken up by the top layer of soil. Furthermore, any rubble that is larger (stones, sticks, leaves) than the plant's stem should be removed. Other than that, follow the 5-step procedure outlined in chapter 4.

As far as hydration goes, the processes are pretty similar to lavender. The marigold plant does accept sandy and dry soil, but will not accept soil that is too hydrated and damp. It is recommended to follow a similar procedure as with lavender when planting the marigold. In pots and containers there should be drainage, and a gravel layer covered with soil when planting helps amazingly well with this. It is important to remember to water the marigolds at the base of the plant, not at the top of the flower. This makes sure no flower damage or rot will start to emerge. Water hoses are generally not preferred either, just use a simple watering can. If the flowers become too heavy during the growth period, consider staking them to a stick or other piece of wood or plastic to keep them in location. However, this extra supportive structure for your herb plant is not always necessary.

To avoid infestations and to encourage growth, cut off dead parts of the plants regularly during the growth seasons (spring and summer) and make sure you use natural pesticides to ward off any unwanted insects or bacteria. A simple insecticidal soap-solution in a spray can could do wonders. Make sure you wash harvested flowers thoroughly to avoid intake of insecticides.

Health Applications

Marigold flower extracts serve a multitude of purposes, and the essential oils really are a great addition to the medicine cabinet in your home. Let's jump right into some of the most essential health-related applications of the marigold plant:

Heals cuts and bruises: The anti-biotic properties in the marigold flower help to quickly heal cuts and bruises. Serving as a blood vessel regrowth accelerator (this sounds super flashy, but studies have shown this is actually the case), skin heals much faster after the application of a little marigold essential oil on the wound.

Fights warts and skin infections: The marigold flower is also strongly anti-inflammatory, which is a helpful characteristic for fighting warts and similar infections. Simple crush the flower and use the juice to apply it to the wart. A similar procedure can be used for other, similar skin infections.

Strengthens the immune system: An interesting effect of using marigold extracts (for example in tea) is that it might help prevent diseases and prevent DNA damage. The essential oils have strong flavonoids and have a strong anti-oxidant effect. Furthermore, the extracts contain considerable amounts of vitamin C, which are needed for the body to function properly.

Slows ageing: The antioxidants help to prevent that the body creates free radicals, which means that the ageing process is slowed down. While there is scientific debate on this topic, it surely cannot be harmful to add some marigold extract to your tea as the side-effects are practically non-existent.

Detoxifies the body: Marigold also is a useful ingredient in detoxification processes. The flower stimulates the lymph system in the body and removes any toxic agents away from your lymphomas. This is also beneficial to the liver, the part of your body responsible to naturally detoxify the body and get rid of unwanted substances.

Helps against bladder infections: The antibiotic and anti-inflammatory nature of the marigold flower helps fight off infections in the bladder and allows the bladder tissue to heal faster.

Eye wash: The wonderful healing components called *lutein*, *zeaxanthin* & *lycopene* are good for the eyes and help prevent any eye infections or diseases. Traditionally, the marigold extracts were used in Ancient Egypt as eyewash to prevent sore red eyes.

Treating colds & flu's: If you have any type of cold, persistent cough or flu, taking a few cups of herbal tea from the marigold flower helps to reduce the irritating symptoms quickly.

Helps prevent bowel diseases & types of cancer: While debate about the effectiveness exists, some people argue that regularly taking some marigold tea might help fight off certain types of cancer. The *lycopene* found in the flower's extract is essential for a healthy prostate, and people suffering from prostate cancer might be benefited by the marigold flower thought limiting the cancer spread and growth. Furthermore, a wide range of lower bowel problems (diarrhea, cramps, IBS, colitis, etc.) can be treated also.

Cures lower-body infections: When using the essential oils in a bath, hemorrhoids can be treated as well. This is also true for other irritations in the lower parts of the body. Examples include the treatment of vaginal infections, bladder infections skin inflammations and possible lower-body other infections. It even helps to ensure a regular period.

Fights rashes and sores: Using a small amount of essential oil on the skin can aid in treatment of skin problems and other types of sores in the upper skin. Take a cloth and infuse it with some marigold oil to treat the skin areas of choice.

Treats arthritis and joint pains: Marigold is also a great product for people suffering from chronic arthritis as well as other types of joint pains. Drinking marigold tea regularly will surely have a beneficial effect for people suffering from these problems. The anti-inflammatory tea reduces any nuisance quickly.

Cosmetic Applications

The anti-bacterial and anti-inflammatory properties of the marigold, in conjunction with their culinary possibilities, make the herb an excellent candidate for a wide variety of cosmetic uses.

The most common application is that in ointments and related skin-care products. The herbal essence of marigold is very useful in acne-treatment and other skin-related problems like rashes and insect bites. Being a potent destroyer of mosquitos, marigold oil can be an ingredient in insect spray. Create your spray by boiling the flowers as well as the leaves, add some soapy water and you have yourself a beautiful organically homemade insecticide. It is also not uncommon to use this (generally harmless) insect spray on the skin of horses to ward of the many mosquitos and flies that they attract during the summertime.

Furthermore, the marigold flower can also be used in homemade shampoos. The properties of marigold allow it to be a good candidate for the production of anti-dandruff shampoo. And people also tend to dip their hair in marigold tea as an alternative. This means that using the extracts from marigold on your head allows you to get rid of annoying dead skin cells on your scalp. Furthermore, it can help prevent the skin from becoming oily.

Potential Dangers

The great thing about marigold is that it has little to no side-effects to it. The fact that the flowers are edible is a clear indication that oral intake of this product is generally safe in lower doses. The flowers and leaves are commonly used in salads and most of the medicinal applications of marigold stem from the use of the flower in herbal tea. While there are almost no side effects, there still are several risk groups that should generally avoid the use of marigold extracts. Women who are either pregnant or breastfeeding should not orally intake the marigold flower, but are free to use the ointments and skin care products. Additionally, it is important to only provide low doses for small children (again, except for the ointments and other skin-related herbal cosmetics).

Also, if a pet accidentally feeds on the flower, make sure there are no signs of poisoning or excess drooling or irritation around the mouth. Generally if a puppy eat the flower it may experience some mild diarrhea or vomiting. The reason that pets have these effects are mainly due to the fact that they lack the enzymes in their body to internally process the plant.

Chapter 7: Rosemary

Rosemary is a popular tastemaker in a wide range of culinary dishes and has a strong fragrance to it. Apart from its culinary value, there are also plenty of health benefits and cosmetic uses to the herb. The evergreen plant is a useful addition to anyone's herb garden as it serves a multitude of practical purposes.

Introduction to Rosemary

Rosemary, specialists in the herbal world like to call it *Rosmarinus officinalis*, is an herb originally found in the Mediterranean European region. Belonging to the mint family, the taste of rosemary is different than expected: a warm, bitter and astringent taste that adds a lot of character to a range of culinary dishes. The beneficial properties of rosemary are lost when too much of the leaves' helpful natural chemical compounds are absorbed by the body.

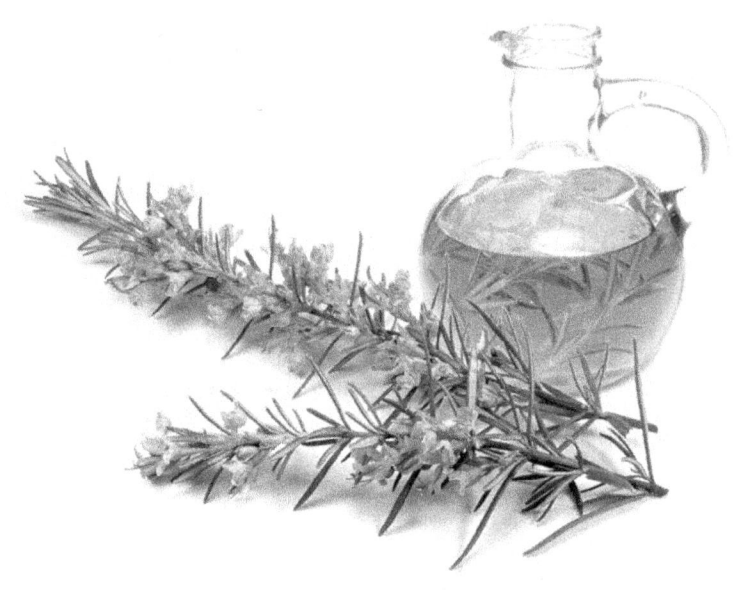

The most common way to solve a multitude of skin problems with this herb is to distill the leaves to a potent essential oil. The essential oil products are also used for several other health-related problems. The richness of the leaves, their nutrients, vitamins and minerals allow the rosemary to be healthy and strongly anti-bacterial and anti-inflammatory. Furthermore, the beneficial aromatic properties in the herb do not only help to give better smell to your garden and home, they also can be used a breath freshener for a naturally clean and fresh breath.

How to Grow

The easiest way to grow rosemary quickly is to grow it from a cutting of another rosemary plant, instead of growing it from the seed. Get several 4 inch (10 cm) cuttings during the late spring and the herb will grow into a fully grown one relatively quickly. Alternatively, buy a complete rosemary plant from your local gardening store or nursery.

When planting cuttings, it is recommended to get a small pot filled with soil (2/3 coarse sand and 1/3 peat moss) and place your cuttings carefully in the soil. Make sure they are placed deep enough and will not easily fall over. Put your pot in a place where the sun shines regularly, but not in full blazing sunlight. In the early stages of growing the cuttings to a well-rooted plant, which is a period of about three weeks, the soil should be watered regularly (daily) and the pot should be placed in a relatively warm spot. The relatively warm temperature can be created by putting the pot in a plastic bag with several holes cut in the top. After three weeks, the roots have formed and the newly created plant is out of its most infant stage, ready to become an adult rosemary herb. The growth process can be sped up if you choose to use rooting powder for the cuttings, which will give your cuttings a solid start in their early life stages.

As soon as the roots have formed, the rosemary plants can start their adult life in the garden or in a bigger, more permanent pot. Luckily for us gardeners, the plant is able to survive most types of weather without a scratch, but thrives best in hot and dry climates. The adapting nature of the herb, however, will allow it to grow pretty much anywhere there is a moderate climate, but it will even grow and survive in places where snow regularly falls. If you decide to grow them in a place where the climate is considered relatively cold, a container or pot is the best option. When the freezing temperatures become too much for regular garden plants to survive in, you are able to move them to a safer location when needed (such as indoors or in a greenhouse). However, you must always make sure with these container growth locations, that the soil can be easily drained so the roots will not get soaked.

For maintenance, there really is a simple procedure that you need to follow. It will generally live off of the rain as it prefers dry soil and warmer climates, but you can water it infrequently when soils get too dry.

Fertilization is not needed, expect for the presence of lime in the soil. Lime is important to regulate the acidity of the soil as well. Furthermore, only prune your plants when they get too big for your liking. The usual moment to prune our plants in in the early spring, as is the case with the other herbs we discussed in this book.

When the herb is ready to be harvested, which can be done all year round, take a pair of scissors and cut off the tops only. This way you will be sure that the rest of the plant will keep growing and serving your needs long-term. It is important to keep your harvested sprigs in a dry and cool place, such as your refrigerator. People tend to prefer the freezer as well for long-terms storage. Put your harvest in air-tight bags, seal them and simply place them in the freezer until you need them. In your freezer the herb will start to become drier and can be kept for multiple months on end. You can either use the rosemary as a culinary ingredient in many types of dishes, or use it around the house or as a health product. Let us take a look at some of the health & cosmetic purposes that this amazing herb has.

Health Applications

The essential oils from rosemary are a potent and very useful ingredient to solve a range of health problems. Be warned that essential oils should always be diluted and are not fit to be taken orally in concentrated form. Let us take a look at some of the most important health applications of the rosemary plant.

Improves mood and reliefs stress: Rosemary is commonly used in aromatherapy. The aromatic benefits of the herb have been scientifically proved to improve overall mood, relieve stress for people who suffer from chronic anxiety or hormonal problems, and helps clearing the mind from thoughts (for example, it can be used during meditation). Aroma from the essential oil is the most effective herbal solution, but the herb itself can do wonders as well.

Boosts memory: Another cognitive benefit to the rosemary herb is to increase retention of memory. Scientists have also seen a positive correlation between rosemary's active ingredients and using the herb for stimulating cognitive capacities in elderly people who suffer from dementia or Alzheimer's disease. It can also be a great memory and focus booster for people seeking to learn large chunks of information in a short period of time. For example, when focusing for a test rosemary can help in the study process.

Strengthens the immune system: There are many properties in the working components of the rosemary's essential oil that can aid the immune system in fighting off harmful intruders in your body. Furthermore, the antioxidant effects of using rosemary will form a second line of defense: preventing oxidation of your body cells and combating the free radicals seeking to cause harm.

Antibacterial and anti-inflammatory: Another element of the herb that aids infighting off diseases are the antibacterial and anti-inflammatory properties. Especially when having bacterial problems in the stomach area, rosemary oil is the ideal candidate to provide a solution.

Blood flow stimulant: The production of red blood cells in the body is stimulated by the active ingredients found in rosemary essence. For the cardiovascular system in the body, this is a huge benefit: your vital organs will have easier access to their much needed oxygen fuel source, allowing the cells to more easily repair themselves and transport their nutrients.

Remedy for upset stomach and gut: One of the most easily upset parts of the body is the stomach, as every part of the day some food or liquid is passing through it. Over centuries and generations, the rosemary plant's primary use was to soothe upset stomachs. Also, the plant has been a helpful soother of any type of gut problem, ranging from diarrhea to bloating and constipation problems.

Pain relief: Another traditional use of the essential oils within the rosemary herb, is the ability to relief pain. Whereas ancient civilizations used it as an ingredient in salve or paste directly on the areas of pain, this natural analgesic is nowadays usually applied in the context of migraine. Again, aromatherapy in combination with applying some essential oil to the temples will help soothe away most of the direct pain experienced.

Improves health of the skin: The anti-inflammatory and detoxification properties of rosemary allow it to be a good skin-health product as well. Both the leaves and the essential oils can be used to improve the quality of the skin and make it look more youthful. However, it is also commonly used to hydrate and oil the surface layers of the skin and make them look healthier.

Cosmetic Applications

The leaf extracts of rosemary serve several purposes in the world of cosmetic products. As a key ingredient, the following types of products make use of the herb for its different beneficial natural characteristics:

Antimicrobial soaps and hand wash: Leaf extract is mainly used for its antimicrobial traits and therefore can be a useful addition in soaps and hand wash products. Any cosmetic product seeking to disinfect can use rosemary for both its smell and ability to fight off bacteria and viruses.

Antioxidant and skin-care products: Mainly serving a role in anti-ageing ointments and related antioxidant sprays, the detoxifying properties of both the leaves and the flower of the herb can be used to improve the skin quality.

Deodorant: The strong natural smell and anti-bacterial properties make for a good combination of traits to produce a quality deodorant. Mainly derived from the essential oils in the flowers, the deodorant ingredients are a good alternative to the traditionally chemically enhanced products on the market today.

Fragrance: It must be apparent right now that the aroma of rosemary is a potent healer and can overall be a good mood enhancer. Therefore, the fragrance (which can be derived from pretty much any oily substance within the plant itself, including the stem and roots) is commonly used in perfumes and other odor-focused cosmetic products.

Potential Dangers

The essential oils of the rosemary herb should never be consumed orally or in a concentrated state. For normal rosemary, the dilution within the plant makes the herb edible without any negative consequences. People who have certain allergies to herbs from the mint family should avoid consumption of this product. However, allergic reactions tend to be mild and non-dangerous overall (and are generally a quite rare occurrence).

As with most of the essential oils, they should not be used by people in certain risk groups, such as pregnant or breastfeeding women. Keep consumption for young children to the bare minimum.

Chapter 8: Aloe Vera

Common by name, the Aloe Vera plant ranks among one of the most commonly used herbs in cosmetic products. However, it also has a wide range of interesting health benefits to it. A small side note being that the liquid goo inside the plant is potentially dangerous. However, adventurous as we are, let us take a closer look at the possibilities of this versatile species.

Introduction to Aloe Vera

Aloe Vera (Latin name: *Aloe barbadenis Mill.*), also known as the 'first aid plant', is a stem-less or short-stemmed succulent or 'fat' plant known for its many medicinal uses. In modern medicinal science some of its medicinal properties are debated. The thick, fleshy leaved plant is however commonly found in many cosmetic products with a wide range of health claims. Also, the plant is loved as a simple house plant by many, simply for its looks and easy maintenance.

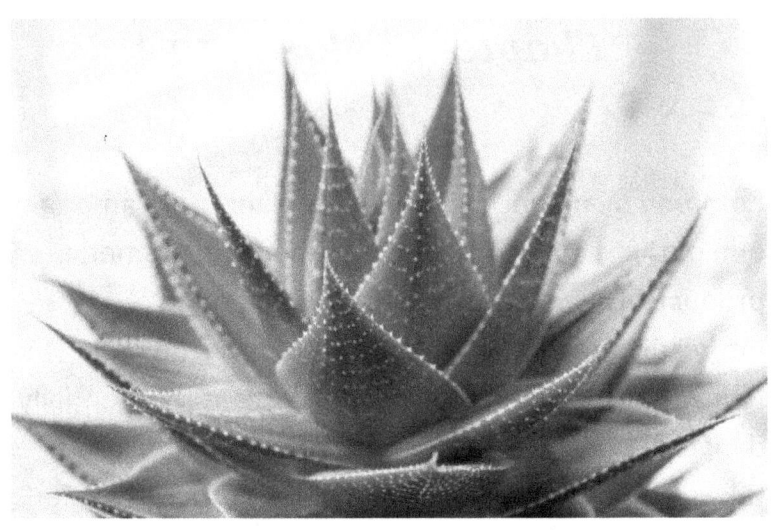

The ancient Egyptians thought the plant was an elixir of life (and called it 'The plant of immortality'), and the ancient Greeks used the plant as a common medicine. Today, you mostly find it in your anti-ageing skin care products or shampoos. The cactus-like plant has been attributed all sorts of wonders, but in the end there are also a lot of people who are skeptical of using it as a medicine. Nevertheless, it is undeniable that the plant is bursting with health-related possibilities. Only looking at the vitamins and minerals within the plant will have you end up with an impressive list of helpful substances. Vitamin A, B1, B2, B6, B12, C, and E are all present. For minerals, the plant contains: aluminum, calcium, calcium-oxalate, chloride, chrome, cobalt, phosphorous, potassium, copper, iron, magnesium, manganese, sodium, selenium, tin and zinc.

Well, and we didn't even discuss the other beneficial ingredients yet. The working components in the plant are an entirely different list of useful substances. Impressive to say the least.

How to Grow

The growth and maintenance process of the Aloe Vera plant is not a very complicated process, which makes this plant one of the ideal candidates to try and grow s your first herb species. It is even possible to grow an entire plant from a single leaf, which is the process that will be explained in this section. However, you could also opt to buy a new plant in your local store.

For the process of growing an entire Aloe Vera plant from a leaf, you will need the following materials to begin with:

- A leaf from the plant itself
- A clay pot with large holes
- Potting soil (and some type of fertilizer)
- Watering hose
- A fragment of broken pottery
- A knife
- A spoon

First we need to prepare the clay pot. It should at least have one large hole in the bottom center to be able to drain excess water. Take the piece of broken pottery and place it over the hole in the bottom, allowing water to flow through but soil to stay inside the pot. Fill the pot with your soil mixture of choice (regular potting soil should be sufficient and provide nutrients to the plant), add fertilizer at your own will. The soil should be filling the pot as high as 1cm to the top of the pot.

Take the Aloe Vera leaf and push it into the soil horizontally. The leaf should still be exposed somewhat. Place the pot into the sunlight and water it. Pill the pot up with water until the edge, then let it drain. Within three to four weeks, you will see the leaf sprouting, but make sure you keep the soil watered regularly.

Assuming you have grown the plant to maturity by placing it in the pot in sunlight and watering it occasionally, you can take out the gel from the leaves after a few months already, all you need is a knife and something to pour the jelly of the leaf into. Cut the leaf lengthwise and make sure you scrape out all the pulp that is left from the leaf. You can do this with a spoon if needed. You have now harvested your first Aloe Vera.

Health Applications

There is a solid reason that the ancient civilizations used the Aloe Vera plant as one of their primary prescriptions towards solving health problems. Despite existing debate in modern medicinal science, there are some proven health applications that are certainly worth it to start growing this plant. Let us take a brief look at the most important beneficial applications.

Anti-everything (except anti-health): The Aloe Vera plant has anti-bacterial, anti-inflammatory, anti-oxidant, anti-biotic, anti-microbial, anti-pyretic (against fevers), anti-septic, anti-fungal and anti-viral properties. That sounds like it is very bad for you, but all these anti-properties are actually amazing for your health! There are a multitude of active ingredients in the plant that help it fight off disease and protect cells. These include phenol, sulfur, urea nitrogen, lupeol, salicyclic acid and cinnamic acid. Their primary functions are to stop the growth of the disease-causing intruders in your body, as well as to fight infections together with the immune system.

Boosts immunity: This brings us the second property of the plant, which is the boost for your body's immune system. The working components in the Aloe Vera plant help stimulate the white blood cells to fight against viruses. Also, the anti-oxidant properties will reduce free radicals in your body and thereby will help slow down the body's ageing process.

Cardiovascular health improvements: It is suggested by some studies that the speed at which oxygen is transported in your blood system is improved when using Aloe Vera extracts. Furthermore, cholesterol can be reduced when taking in the (diluted and mixed!) juice of the plant.

Acceleration of burn healing: We are talking about skin burns here, to be precise. We should not only apply cold water to the burned area, but also some Aloe Vera essence in order to speed up the healing process of the skin. This is also the case for bug bites, abrasions, psoriasis and related skin issues. It provides immediate pain relief and provides an instant soothing affect when rubbing some essence on the burned area of the skin. Furthermore, it will hydrate and moisturize the skin again which hallows the pores to open and the blood to flow better.

Treats mouth ulcers: Those painful spots you sometimes have in your mouth are called mouth ulcers (or alternatively: canker sores). They can be really painful and annoying, especially when eating food or brushing your teeth. And you guessed it right, mouth ulcers can be treated using Aloe Vera treatment. The size of the ulcers has proven to reduce when applying the herb to the painful spots. Another scientific study found that the gel extracts from the plant were able to reduce the pain from these tiny sores in your mouth.

Treats constipation: Using Aloe Vera can really mess with your digestive system, which is one of the primary risks of using the plant for medicinal use. However, it also means that any type of constipation will be solved with a quick race to the toilet after using the extracts from this plant. The essential component that should be used this time is not the gel (which should not be indigested orally!), but the latex, which is the sticky and yellow-colored residue located under the leaf skins of the plant. The *aloin*, which is the working component in this case, is strongly laxative and can really 'blast away' some of your digestive problems.

Lowers blood sugar levels for diabetics (unconfirmed): While unconfirmed by medicinal science, some studies suggest a correlation between lower blood sugar levels. Aloe Vera has traditionally been used as a remedy against diabetes, but the effects are hard to prove. Aloe Vera is supposedly helpful to enhance the sensitivity of the insulin in your body, thereby aiding the overall regulation of the blood sugar levels in your entire body.

Cosmetic Applications

There is a very wide range of cosmetic products which use Aloe Vera in some way shape or form as a main working ingredient in their products. This section will cover the most important product groups which you will be benefited from the plant in a cosmetic sense.

Skin products: The main use of Aloe Vera is for use on the skin. The liquid substance within the leaves of the plant are great natural replacements for many types of skin care products. By making your own ointments with Aloe Vera, you can make products that help improve skin elasticity and reduce wrinkles. The detoxifying properties (the many different working components within the plant itself) will eventually make the skin look younger. The skin will get more elastic and flexible, because the working components within the plant help with the repair of collagen and elastin (important for a youthful and flexible skin). Aloe Vera is mostly water, which will also hydrate, soften and soothe the skin whilst at the same time helping the overall skin blood flow and strength as well as synthesis of the skin tissue.

Mouth and dental: Another common product using Aloe Vera is mouthwash. Simply as pure juice, the natural product seemed just as effective at removing bacteria from the mouth as regular mouthwash products. The product was able to effectively reduce the amount of dental plaque in the mouth, which is the primary cause of dental problems and tooth caveats. Tooth decay, as well as gum problems, are also reduced when using the Aloe Vera 'goo' as an alternative to the normal mouthwash made from a substance called *chlorhexidine*. For the same reasons as dental plaque removal, the working substances will also quickly get rid of mouth ulcers (also known as canker sores), which are painful sores that will often appear in the gum of the mouth.

Bites and burns: Heal rashes and regular skin infections as well as wounds and bruises with the Aloe Vera plant with ease. The plant is astringent, which means that it will cause certain skin contractions when applied. This particular effect is very helpful in the process of healing skin wounds or burns. It will instantly reduce bleeding from minor wounds and cuts, as well as helping to oxidize the skin quickly. This also means that applying Aloe Vera to minor bruises and burns will give instant pain relief. This certainly includes sunburns, so feel free to experiment with creating some homemade after-sun products. When having a strong itch or bug bite pain, Aloe Vera will help as well because of the earlier mentioned skin contractions it causes. The helping process is sped up tremendously and you will have some relief because of the cold hydrated Aloe Vera gel on your skin as well.

Potential Dangers

Do not ingest the inside liquid substance of the Aloe Vera plant directly! Oral use of the liquid can be very dangerous to your health. The substance is officially labeled as carcinogenic and can cause serious harm in large amounts accumulating into the body. If you have accidentally taken in a significant amount of the liquid goo inside the plant, please consult a doctor immediately.

Another important thing to mention is the latex of the plant, which can be possibility just as dangerous because of its effects on the digestive system. High doses of this product should not be used at ALL times, and the use in small doses is possibly unsafe for certain groups of people.

You should avoid Aloe Vera products all together when pregnant or breastfeeding, or when you are a child below the age of 12. People with diabetes should continuously monitor their blood sugar levels when using the plant to ensure their levels will not get too low. When you have Crohn's disease, ulcerative colitis, or obstruction, it is best to avoid doses of the latex products. Also, when you have hemorrhoids, kidney problems or two weeks before surgery, it is best to avoid the latex products of the Aloe Vera plant.

Chapter 9: Lemon Balm

As the name of this common herbal species suggests, lemon balm is an odorous herb (smelling like, well, lemons) with a multitude of beneficial possibilities. Easy to grow, lemon balm can provide solutions you would not have imagined by the looks of the species.

Introduction to Lemon Balm

This herb from the mint family is officially called *Melissa officinalis*. Whilst the herb is native to the warmer European regions, Northern Africa and parts of Asia, it is commonly used throughout the world, mainly for its many culinary and medicinal purposes and benefits. It does have flowers, but we are primarily looking for the beneficial characteristics of the leaves of the lemon balm herb.

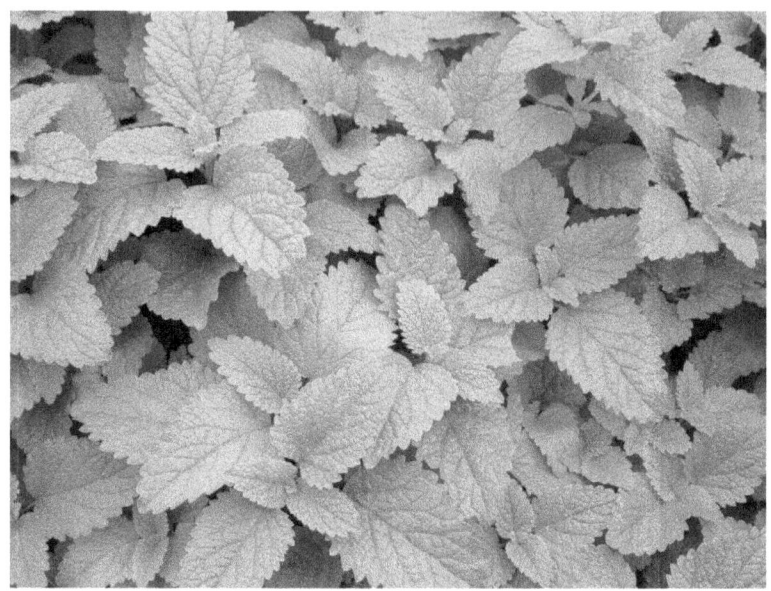

Lemon balm is a plant that will grow the fastest of all the plants described in this book. The plant is easy to grow and can adapt to many types of circumstances, and will sprout throughout your entire herb garden if you are not careful. Therefore, it is quite important to designate a specific area to this specific herb to avoid unwanted spread of the herb throughout your garden. However useful the plant itself can be, too much of it can become quite a nuisance, so keep the growth potential in mind when planting this herb. A good tip is to remove the flowers from the plant once they start sprouting in order to avoid further unwanted spread.

In food, lemon balm is an excellent flavoring. It is mainly used in ice creams and herbal teas, but can serve as a tastemaker in many more dishes. Generally, using the herb culinary is done in combination with fruits or candy. So for the sweet tooth out there, this herb is definitely for you. And it might help you out with some medicinal problems as well, which we will talk about in a bit...

How to Grow

Lemon balm is a perennial plant, meaning that it can grow more than one season. It will generally grow in all types of soil, but prefers clay or sand-type soils that have little hydration to them. It is therefore quite logical that the plant prefers a drier climate over a wet one. The soil to put the lemon balm in can even be a little acidic: between 6.0 and 7.5 pH level is fine for this particular herb. It will grow up to 18 inches in height (45cm) on average.

When planting seedlings, the best moment to do this is in early spring. Start by growing a few seedlings in a pot indoors (around 7 weeks before the last frost), and place the pot near a space with natural sunlight. Alternatively, you could place seeds on top of the soil after the last frosty day in the early spring. Lemon balm will always find a way to sprout, no need to worry about that. It is more a matter of keeping the plant under control once it starts growing, as it can quite rapidly become a nuisance.

When placing your seedlings in the garden when they grow up, make sure to place them a little apart (roughly 15 inches or 38 centimeters). The plant will thrive in relatively dry soils in the full sun, or when there is a partial shady area. It is recommended to use a pot or container away from other, more vulnerable species of plants or herbs, since the proliferation and overall growth of the seedlings can happen quite rapidly. Ensure that you water them not too much, and the plant will have no trouble growing by itself. Remove the flowers before they open to reduce the possibility of the plant spreading too quickly in your garden.

Growth time between seedlings and harvesting is short, roughly 10 weeks. When the plant is fully grown you can harvest it by removing the leaves. Pick them individually or remove entire branches, depending on how large you want to keep the rest of the plant. The harvest time can be considered as 'year-round' (except in wintertime). After taking the leaves, they can be easily stored.

Storing your leaves is a simple process, simply dry your leaves in a dark and relatively cool place. Store them for example in an airtight glass or plastic container. The leaves can be stored for up to one year without any type of issue. Use a distiller to get the most out of the essential oil harvest, as described earlier in this book for other herbal species. It is important to note that the essential oils from the lemon balm is created from the flowers, which can be distilled into a beautiful oil substance. The essential oils themselves can be used for a multitude of purposes, which we will discuss in the following sections.

Health Applications

There are numerous health benefits attributed to the lemon balm herb, more specifically the health benefits from the different working components within the leaves of the plant itself. Let us briefly go over some of the most important medicinal purposes of lemon balm.

Soothing and calming to the mind: Often used as part of aromatherapy, the scent of lemon balm is very helpful in creating an indoors environment that is very calming and soothing to the mind. Just the aroma itself from the concentrated essential oil will bring you into a state of calmness, which is generally experienced as pleasant by people using it as part of therapy. Generally, people experiencing the scent of the herb are reported to have gotten a more positive overall mood.

Improves the possibility of restful sleep: Connected to the previous point, the calming and soothing characteristics of the herb will help you feel well-rested and allow you to have a better and deeper sleep overall. The working components within the lemon balm allow you to lower the overall brain activity during the peaceful state of mind you are in whilst sleeping. Taken in the form of supplements, lemon balm can be indigested without problems, as it is an edible plant. Scientific studies have proven that especially women during menopause can benefit from these supplements in order to improve their sleep ritual.

Detoxifies the body and supports the liver: As we all might have learned in biology class at some point, the liver is the primary organ in the body for removing toxins. Supporting this organ in any way possible will therefore be helpful in getting rid of unwanted 'waste' inside your body – exactly what lemon balm is a great help for. It will aid your liver in the production of the anti-oxidants with the most appealing names ever: *gluthathione* and *superoxide dismutase*. Furthermore, the natural detox process over time will damage your liver cells: lemon balm can slow down this (normal) ageing process through its natural anti-oxidant properties, thus allowing your liver to, in essence, extent its lifespan. Especially recommendable for people with high alcohol consumption or other liver-damaging diets.

Helps regulate blood sugar levels: Another aspect of the body that can wear down over time due to your diet (as well as genetic traits), is related to your blood sugar levels. Diabetes is one of the most commonly found diseases in Americanized countries, and regulating your blood sugar level is a daily practice for people suffering from this chronic disease. Lemon balm will help with the regulation of the natural blood sugar levels in your body. When consuming the herb your body's insulin resistance will be reduced and therefore a positive effect can be seen for the regulation of your overall blood sugar level, scientific studies have found.

Protects cells in your brain: Well, might seem like it is a little far-fetched, but it is actually true that lemon balm will stop the brain from becoming damaged. The detoxifying properties of the lemon balm will ward of free radical and help your brain to survive the free radicals-attack. The working component here is called *eugenol*, a substance that neutralizes free radicals and protect the brain tissue from being damaged. Some components in lemon balm (such as *rosemarinic acid*) have even been used to treat victims of a stroke.

Cosmetic Applications

The world of cosmetics is very familiar with the lemon balm herb, as it is used in many types of skin care products. The soothing effect the herb has on the skin, together with the detoxifying effects, allows it to be a perfect candidate within a lot of skin-related products, just as is the case with a lot of herbs within the mint family. Let us look at some of the most common groups of cosmetics where lemon balm is a common ingredient, which can be easily made within your home as well with some basic ingredients.

Natural skincare: Lemon balm improves skin quality and makes skin look younger, mainly because of the working components in the essential oils and leaves that have anti-ageing properties. Fighting off free radicals in the body (which are naturally occurring) is a highly sought after trait in the skin-care industry. You can easily make your own homemade organic skin-care product that improves the youth and hydration of the skin. Also, the scent of the lemon balm will make the plant a good candidate within deodorants and similar products, mainly because of the benefits to the skin and the strong odor of the essential oil.

Make a glycerite for calmness: A glycerite is a fluid extract that is used to collect the herbal plant's glycerin. This product will help you reduce stress and improve your overall feeling of calmness. Gather some fresh lemon balm leaves and put them in a glass jar. Cover the leaves with 3 parts vegetable glycerite (which can be bought in most large supermarket chain stores, or alternatively online. I prefer to use a soy glycerite) and one part water. Close the jar air-tight and store it in a dark, cool place for up to 4 weeks. Consume ½ to 1 teaspoon of the substance to ensure calmness of mind and instant stress-relief. It is recommended to store the jar in the refrigerator after the period of 4 weeks.

Bathing product: Get a simple bag that allows water to get through. Fill the small bag with flower petals from a rose and leaves from the lemon balm herb. Hang it from the spigot in your bath and allow the water to flow through the bag s your bath fills up. Guaranteed that you will enjoy your amazing herbal bath water. Great for both skin and calmness of mind.

Potential Dangers

The lemon balm herb is an edible plant, is considered non-toxic and the herb is generally not irritating, thus the potential dangers are limited. Mainly, using the essential oils in concentrated form has the greatest danger potential.

As with most herbal species, the lemon balm oil should never be used by pregnant or breastfeeding women. The hormonal balance can be affected which will have consequences for the baby. For children, low doses for medicinal or cosmetic use are acceptable, but should be avoided under the age of 12 if possible.

Another interesting effect are the mild sedative properties of lemon balm essential oil. It is recommended to not use the oil when operating any type of dangerous equipment or machinery, and to not use the oil when doing a task that requires a high focus.

While the sedative effects wear off quite rapidly and are overall not very noticeable in normal healthy humans, the precautionary principle should be number one here. Don't take any unnecessary risks and simply do not use dangerous tools or equipment after using lemon balm oil products.

Chapter 10: Basil

We conclude our list of herbal plants by looking at one of my favorite species, which is the famous basil. Commonly used in the kitchen where it is referred to as 'the king of herbs', this culinary wonder has a lot of other potentially beneficial traits to it in the medicinal and cosmetic world.

Introduction to Basil

Basil, also referred to as Thai or sweet basil, sometimes even called 'Saint Joseph's Wort', is an herbal plant that belongs to the mint family. Its scientific Latin name is *Ocimum basilicum*. Used for over 5000 years, the plant is native to India, Afghanistan and Pakistan. It has been spreading mainly for its distinct taste, and therefore used in many types of different food dishes.

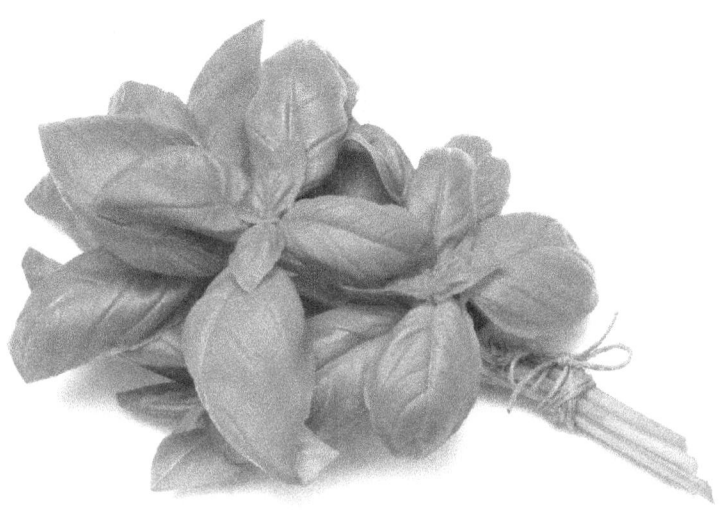

Some interesting observations from historical herbalists really describe the character of this plant quite well. For example, herbalist John Gerard spoke about how those stung by a scorpion would feel no pain after eating some basil. Another observation was that because of the healing powers, some Mexican tribes believed that the herb would cleanse them of evil spirits. The plant has a long track-record of being associated with the afterlife and death itself.

The herb is commonly planted on graves, such as is common practice on the altars of the Greek Orthodox churches. Jewish lore spoke of the strength that the plant provided the people during the fasting period, simply by holding some basil leaves in the hand. An interesting history for a multi-purpose gift from nature.

How to Grow

When starting from the seed, growing basil is a relatively straight-forward process, but it does take some time and effort. First of all, choose your favorite species of basil as there are many types and varieties which can be used. Every single species has their own characteristics, smells and flavors. Some examples include Lemon basil (lemon taste), Cinnamon basil (sweet with fragrant flowers), Purple basil (mainly decorative, so not preferred when using it in a practical sense), Thai basil (sweet anise-like scent and spicy flavors), or Greek basil (only for advanced growers, difficult plant).

As with most plants, when planting seedlings, the best moment to go about doing this is in early spring. Start by growing a few seedlings in a pot indoors (around 4 to 6 weeks before the last frost), and place the pot near a space with natural sunlight. It is important to place the seedlings in warm air and sun, as these are the optimal growing conditions for our baby basil sprouts. What we want to do is to prepare our seed pots or containers with a special soil mixture of peat, perlite and vermiculite (all equal parts). Fill the pot or container up to about 1 inch from the top, and press the soil downwards to remove any excess air. Pour water into the soil mixture and get your basil seeds ready.

Each pot or container needs exactly two seeds. Place them in a tiny hole and put soil over them. Then continue to put some see-through thin kitchen wrap (plastic) over the pots to assure the soil will remain moist as your seedlings grow. Put the pots in the sun near a window, water twice a day it is recommended to remove the plastic before watering, otherwise we are watering plastic and not the soil).When the sprouts become visible after a few days it is time to remove our plastic cover. Watering should remain twice a day as we did before the sprouts emerged. Make sure the soil stays moist throughout the day. When the plants are a few inches, its transportation time to a larger pot and into the outside garden. Do this once two leave sets have been formed and make sure to put them in a place where the sun shines.

The soil from the pot should be able to drain as well, so ensure there is at least one hole in the pot or container you place the plants in. Place your small basil plants 6 inches (15cm) apart, so make sure that when you place multiple plants in the same container that your soil area is large enough. Keep the soil damp, but not soaked, water with care throughout the lifetime of the plant. Water them once a day in the morning, preferably. Make sure your plant lives in an environment that is generally warmer than 50 degrees Fahrenheit (10 degrees Celsius). Frostbite is a serious problem for basil, we want to keep our plants from getting too cold outside.

When the flowers start to emerge, we want to remove those as soon as they pop up. This is to ensure the taste will remain good. When flowers will stay on the basil, the hormonal changes within the plant will start to alter the plant. Also, flower growth reduces the ability for the plant to grow the leaves (and the leaves are what we will need for our harvest). Check regularly that no molds or insects start nesting themselves in or on the plants. Japanese beetles love hanging out on basil, we want to keep those creatures away from our precious plants. If mod grows on the plants, weed out some plants to ensure they get enough sunlight. Mold is often a side-effect of lack of sunlight over plants being grown too close together. Prune regularly when the basil grows too close together.

The time is right for harvesting when the plants grow too large or when they have reached a reasonable height. What we want to do is to pinch off the two pairs of basil leaves at the top of the plant (never at the base). We want to make sure when pruning and cutting plant that we leave the growth potential for the smaller leaves intact. When you feel like you have removed enough leaves, clean them with water and store them in the refrigerator (or use the fresh leaves immediately). Long-term storage of leaves is possible in the freezer, but to ensure quality make a puree from them first. They will remain usable for months. Alternatively dry them and store them in a cold and dark place: this is preferred for most medicinal uses. The basil leaves are a great ingredient in many dishes, so consuming them is a great idea as well. However, we mainly are looking for the leaves in a context of health improvements.

Health Applications

Multiple medicinal applications characterize the basil plant. The most important applications of the herb are discussed below. The key medicinal parts of the plant include the leaves, flowering tops and the essential oil. It is even inhaled with steam to relieve nasal congestions. Please note that these medicinal purposes should always be used in a safe context – consult the final section of this chapter for potential dangers when using the plant as a medicinal resource.

Treats fevers and common colds: Basil leaves have an abundance of healing properties, most of which can be attributed to phytonutrients and the essential oils extracted from the plant. The working components will aid in healing dengue and malarial fevers, as well a regular fevers. Furthermore, the natural disinfectants of the plant will help protect against possible bacterial or viral infections in the body. This also means that basil leaves are useful to treat the common cold and will aid you in healing faster. For treatment of the common cold, simply brew a tea from dried basil leaves, or chew on some fresh leaves instead (don't worry, basil is an edible plant used in many food dishes). For something stronger like a heavy fever, a more serious brew might be helpful. The following treatment is recommended:

Ingredients:

- 0.5 liters of water
- Sugar
- Milk
- Powdered cardamom
- Fresh or dried basil leaves

How to make the brew:

Mix the 0.5 liters of water with some sugar and milk to taste. Add the leaves to the mixture and slowly stir the powdered cardamom into the mixture as well. Boil this brew and serve it to the patient every three hours during the fever, until the patients core temperature has lowered again.

Treats coughs and sore throat: When making herbal tea from the leaves of the basil plant, the anti-bacterial and anti-viral properties will help fight the infections in throats and lungs. When suffering from a heavy cough or simply when having a sore or infected throat, make some herbal tea and your problems will be gone after a few cups of this healthy and delicious natural drink. Alternatively, use a steam bath based on basil leaves. Take one tablespoon for every two cups of water. Put the heated mixture in a large pot and cover your head with a towel, breathing in the steam for roughly 10 minutes for instant relief.

Vomiting relief provider: For people that suffer from high-frequency vomiting, a basil mixture will help provide relief and reduce the vomiting problems. The recommended basil-based solution is a simple mixture of basil leaves and ginger juice and some honey for sweetness. Dilute the mixture with some water if needed and you will have created a helpful natural remedy against vomiting problems.

Improves focus and reliefs stress: It's time to chew basil leaves again – when you chew on a dozen basil leaves twice a day, your stress-levels will rapidly drop, your blood will be purified and your mind and focus will be improved. Basil leaves are a perfect anti-stress and mind-enhancing agent and they will actively alter your cardiovascular system, neurological system and hormonal system for the better.

Beneficial to the eyes: Not only carrots are good for your eyes, basil leaves will aid your eyes as well. The herb contains an abundance of Vitamin A, which is very good for the eyes. Washing your eyes with basil leave-based substance your overall visual health will be improved as it prevents stress in the eye sockets, swelling, infections, sore eyes, night blindness, inflammations and conjunctivitis. Also, chewing on basil leaves regularly will help as a preventive measure against cataracts, deterioration of vision as well as glaucoma.

Treats kidney stones: A very painful ordeal is having to deal with kidney stones. Basil juice might help you with this very painful kidney problem over time. During a period of 6 months, take some basil leaf juice together with honey to be able to expel those annoying kidney stones from your urinal tract. A long-term but certainly worthwhile health solution.

Headache relief: Many people also use a basil-based steam bath for their face. Simply use dried basil leaves and hot water and a towel for this process. One tablespoon for every two cups of water will be sufficient. Put the heated mixture in a large pot and cover your head with a towel, taking up the steam with your face for about 10 minutes. Breathing in the steam is the most effective method here. This will aid with instant relief of most types of headaches, as well as helping to reduce the common cold or any type of painful throat sores.

Beneficial to the heart and lungs: Respiratory and heart diseases can be treated and prevented with basil as well. Either basil tea or the earlier mentioned mixture of ginger juice, basil juice and honey will aid you in this process. The mixture is a natural treatment for bronchitis, coughs and colds, asthma and other lung-related problems. Basil also purifies and detoxifies the blood, which in turn will aid with the improvement of the cardiovascular health in your body.

Treats skin infections and ringworms: Anti-bacterial, anti-fungal and anti-inflammatory properties within the basil leaves will help fight off bacterial growth related to skin infections. When applied on the skin, a mixture of 250 grams of basil leaves with sesame oil and some water will help in the process of treating most types of skin problems. The mixture can be applied to the area where the problem persists. Also, mix lemon juice and basil leaves with some water to ward off and fight ringworms that have invaded your body.

Cosmetic Applications

As with most of the herbs discussed in this book, there is a wide range of practical applications to be considered. Next to all the health benefits, there are also multiple uses in the world of cosmetics that can make for some great helpful products. These are certainly worth considering when you take your herbal garden to the next level, or simply are interested in the fine art of creating organically produced, homemade cosmetics.

Skin care products: Basil leave extracts are very good for the rejuvenation of the skin and for treating several skin-related problems. The anti-bacterial and anti-inflammatory nature of the plant will help the skin to become healthy and look younger. Treatments are twofold: either through consuming the basil leaves or by applying a basil-leaf based skin paste.

As a preventive measure, basil leaves are great to ward off acne problems or pimples. This is mainly attributed to the toxins that are removed from the bloodstream after consuming sufficient amounts of the herb itself. However, when acne or other skin surface problems start to emerge, applying a basil-based paste will help reducing the inflammation as well. Mix with rose water, sandalwood or neem paste to get the most optimal skin recovery effect.

Other skin-related improvements in the face include the benefits to facial skin and then neck skin in general. Rubbing the dried leaves on your face and neck will give your skin a young and fresh look for facial and neck skin. Also, it prevents blackheads to appear on the nose. If you suffer from Vitiligo (white patches of skin), these can be treated as well with the dried leaves.

Get rid of stings and bug bites by chewing basil leaves or applying basil leave oils directly from the leaf onto the painful or itchy area. This will provide instant relief for the skin. Additionally, applying the basil leave juice directly to the skin will help to get rid of any type of sub-skin venom.

Hair products: The basil's essential oil can be used as an ingredient in shampoos or hair gels. Basil rejuvenates the hair follicles and allows the hair shaft to be strengthened. Also, it will prevent possible hair loss due to removing itchiness and sweatiness from the scalp.

The anti-ageing properties of the working components in basil supposedly will also reduce the speed at which grey hairs will emerge. The basil plant is reported to have antioxidants in them, which are helpful in fighting off free radicals that are detrimental to the hairs.

Mouth products: Several health treatments involve chewing on basil leaves to improve the cardiovascular system, among other things. However, a useful side-effect of chewing the leaves is that it will get rid of bad breath and improve dental health. It is a perfect natural substitute to chewing gums, toothpastes and other dental products that are anti-bacterial in nature. For the toothpaste, dried and powdered leaves and mustard oil make a great basic set of ingredients. This product will remove plaque and strengthen the gum health.

Another interesting use of chewing basil leaves is that it is useful for trying to quit smoking. Smoking clearly is a habit that is difficult to stop solely by your own motivation and mental power, but chewing on basil leaves might help get rid of the habit of smoking over time, possibly more so than the nicotine patches you can buy in your local supermarket or pharmacy. It will replace the need for a cigarette with the need to chew on some leaves, which is actually a healthy habit that will improve both heart and lungs over time.

Potential Dangers

It is important that the essential oils of the basil plant should not be used during pregnancy or during breastfeeding periods. This is the case for both internal and external use, as it might be harmful to the child.

Children should generally stay away from using basil from medicinal purposes. Especially infants are at risk when being exposed to the plant. Nevertheless, do not be afraid when using basil as a tastemaker in your dishes: normal cooking amounts are too little to be harmful. Only the concentrated essential oil products should be avoided, generally.

For people who suffer from diabetes, medicinal use the herb can be harmful in larger amounts. The active components in basil can interfere with the required medicine for diabetics. So to be sure, if you have diabetes, do not use the plant for any type of medicinal purpose. Consult your medical assistant and ask them for what purposes the basil herb can be used, as not all uses are necessarily dangerous. Furthermore, a normal culinary use should not be harmful to diabetics.

Chapter 11: Parting Words

Growing and nursing an herbal garden can be a lengthy but very rewarding process. All the way from the gardening and maintenance of your herbs, down to the harvesting and practical application: naturally produced herbal medicinal solutions are certainly a work of effort. However, being able to work with natural products in the comfort of your own home garden is a unique worthwhile process. After all, growing your own herbal garden is a process of personal development and learning as well. The skills taught in the process are invaluable and can be passed down to many other like-minded people eager to learn about our natural world and its practical uses and applications.

In the process of setting up and taking care of your own natural health and cosmetic solutions, you will be able to provide for others in a self-sufficient manner. People seeking to live off the grid and teach themselves unique valuable skills about the uses of herbal plants in order to attain this self-sufficiency are sure to see the value in the information provided in this book. Also, those seeking to find medical solutions that differentiate from the traditional pharmaceutical world will be more than welcoming of these natural solutions.

As a closing note, I wish to thank you for taking the time to read *Homegrown Medicinal Herbs*. Through the course of this book, we have showed you the many possible medicinal and cosmetic applications of several well-known species of herbal plants, gave an introduction on how to grow these herbs in your own garden or homestead, as well as the potential dangers that could result from using these herbs for specific purposes. We opened your world to the possibilities of herbalism and its many uses and we have brought you one step closer to complete self-sufficiency in your daily life. Please take the lessons from this book and apply them to the real world! Starting an herbal garden is not complicated at all. And you will find great joy in the process for sure.

Thank you for taking the time to read this introductory book to homegrown medicinal herbs. If you would like to keep in touch with me and receive my future books for free, you can follow me on Facebook or Twitter. Simply type in my author name and you will find me. I always love to keep my audience informed. Thanks!

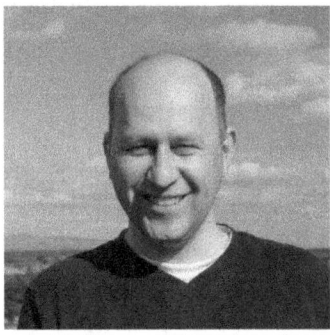

William Walsworth

Author, biologist & sustainable living expert